DIFFICULT TO KILL:

Master the mindset to augment your years

BY

Catherine J. Burns

Table of contents

DESCRIPTION

A ton of things can be purchased in this world, however, your well-being isn't one of them. The main individual who can accomplish ideal well-being will invest the effort. To make the most out of your single opportunity on the planet, you want to turn into an expert on the five pillars of health:

Pillar 1: Healthy food

Pillar 2: Movement

Pillar 3: Sleep

Pillar 4: Connection

Pillar 5: Exercise

Difficult To Kill will give you a guide that will assist you with dominating those five support points, making you truly, intellectually, and profoundly solid. A misstep pursued at least a few times is a decision. Decided to be difficult To Kill.

INTRODUCTION

From the moment we are conceived, the main assurance in life is death. This might seem like a cruel reality, however as an OBGYN, it's something I contemplate each time I deliver a child. I also ponder the potential outcomes of who they will become-what they will accomplish and the effect they will leave on the world.

Everybody leaves inheritance when we're presently not here. An inheritance that recounts the lives we contacted during our lifespan. Significance is the capacity to motivate individuals around you. I need to move you so you can motivate others. The central issue is "How incredible would you say you are?

The assurance of death makes our lifespan so valuable. It is an example I learned after a horrible life-altering situation that turned into the impetus to change for me and my friends and family. It is the reason each one requires to make a quality life and why I need to give you the expertise to make that existence with anything that time you are given. All things considered, energy is our most significant resource, and the most effective way to boost them is by becoming somebody difficult to kill.

There are five pillars of well-being expected to accomplish a quality life and become difficult to kill; healthy food, movement, exercise, connection and sleep. Every one of the pillars cooperates. You can't disregard one for the other.

I will give point-by-point clarification about every pillars of well-being with the goal that you will acquire a top to bottom information on every one of them and how to integrate them into your own life.

Being difficult to kill is something other than fighting off ailment or illnesses. It's awakening every day with a deep longing to need the existence you have and all that it envelops.

Being difficult to kill isn't ideal for everyone, it's a way of life frequently lived on the edges.

Turning out to be difficult to kill is certainly not a handy solution that works out coincidentally. It's a long-lasting mindset, and the quickest method for arriving is gradual.

CHAPTER ONE

Youth is lost on the youthful

Adulthood puts expectations on us and tests our capacities in some cases. It tends to be very difficult because we are not kids who have grown-ups to do the reasoning and a large portion of the work. Also, nobody truly showed us as kids what adulthood would be like. What's the general purpose of adulthood? Is it anything but an inconvenience to develop into adulthood? No, this article makes sense of being a grown-up.

Being a grown-up is very difficult, yet the entire idea of it is TAKING RESPONSIBILITY. The facts confirm that you'll take care of bills, try sincerely and shrewdly, and have high points and low points. It is likewise a fact that it won't generally be ruddy, and your monetary choices must be made by you. You want to find a consistent line of work. You'd be answerable for your clothing, cook your feasts, and some more.

Yet, it's anything but a weakness to assume liability. All things being equal, it's a valuable chance to demonstrate to life that you're not unremarkable, and are fit for battling your direction through to make a big deal about your life. It's likewise a method for kicking your difficulties in the butt by showing that your fantasies merit battling for.

Be that as it may, it gets intense and depleting in some cases. Here is a speedy one, even with difficulties, could you rather continue up or surrender? It is smarter to get a sense of ownership of your life and battle your direction through.

I extol every individual who is a grown-up and is endeavoring to make it paying little mind to how extreme it gets now and then. Challenges come at minutes in your day-to-day existence where you can capitalize on possibilities inside you and make your fantasies a reality. It is a period where you learn, forget, and relearn. It is a stage where you fabricate reasonable and beneficial associations with individuals. It is a timeframe where you track down affection, where you learn to balance. It is a period when you ought to mean to get better in your funds in a genuine way. On the off chance that you do this, your fantasy about giving yourself a superior life wouldn't stay a fantasy for eternity.

Adulthood is certainly a rollercoaster, however, that's the short and long of it right? There will constantly be great times, terrible times, victories, and disappointments. We will not necessarily in all cases have high highs; life could happen now and again. There's dependably an appearance of lows regardless of how high and professional things might appear.

Certainly, it could turn out intense. Some of the time you'd consider stopping since you figure you probably won't make due. However, prepare to have your mind blown. You don't need to stop. In five years to come, in 10 years to come, you'll recall that you didn't surrender, and you'll congratulate yourself. You will say thanks to yourself for that strong move toward staying simultaneously, and not yield to dread of the difficulties that come in your direction.

Being a grown-up is testing, however not a drawback. Very few grown-ups figure out this. They have surrendered to the tension that difficulties bring. They have some unacceptable mindset of how they ought to be dealt with and have chosen to label adulthood as a trick.

Does this make things any better? No, it doesn't. This thought that adulthood is a trick breeds unremarkableness. Then you begin to see these individuals abandoning their fantasies to be better individuals and become something else for them as well as their reality. At the point when you begin inviting the possibility that adulthood is only a trick, you'd quit pushing and begin making do with less.

Getting out of your usual range of familiarity will then become something you won't do.

The Struggle is Real

Every day we are confronted with circumstances that are not so great. We get through battles in our marriage, kinships, and occupations. Battles are a piece of life, yet they don't need to characterize it.

There's an inquiry we toss around that I bet implies significantly more than we would anticipate. How often per week — or a day! — are you inquired,

"How are you?"

Let's be real, the response I hear and give most is something like . . . "fine" or "occupied yet great!" It's kind of the socially satisfactory response, isn't that so?

A companion posed this inquiry simply this week as I strolled into work. I was performing multiple tasks as expected while kneeing somewhere down in a PDA discussion about one more issue. I didn't respond to her, since, in such a case that I did — on the off chance that I truly halted and replied — I could have begun crying, not too far off on the spot. My lips shaped "fine" when in actuality, I was everything except — to some degree at that time. Furthermore, life doesn't necessarily in all cases stop to the point of offering a genuine response.

However, "fine" is the socially satisfactory response since it works . . . or on the other hand right?

We are battling, to various degrees and intricacy levels, every single day. The battle is genuine, and when you include both the little and enormous everyday battles, it's straightforward why this hashtag virtual entertainment rockstar exists — north of 3 million deep at #thestruggleisreal.

Yet, on the off chance that we dig somewhat more profound into this normal objection, we could find a considerably more vile root — and genuine assistance toward opportunity.

I composed this book since I know how genuine the battle is — and I believe that we should find the genuine wellspring of the solution to these deep-rooted issues. I would like to take perusers through an excursion into this hole between our "fine and dandy" day-to-day routines and the genuinely great lives we are looking for and are eager for. To offer the expectation that we can carry on with the best life we can, this side of paradise.

That's right, the battle is certainly genuine. Be that as it may, the battle can likewise begin the story. It can propel us to change our lives into another story. The battles can lead us to another wellspring of trust and opportunity — and in some way or another, even the most terrible of life can turn into a position of solidarity and development. The battle is genuine. Also, the battle can be great.

A life with purpose and passion

The Two words, 'purpose' and 'passion', consistently appeared to be so colossal, so distant, so unreachable for so many years and I would deliver a conjecture that that is how you would portray them as well! Indeed, fortunately finding your motivation and enthusiasm in life isn't generally so troublesome as we would have been persuaded to think. It's quite straightforward…

To this end, many individuals don't accept that they've tracked down it! Since they have this thought in their mind that when they, at last, find the sacred goal all that will make sense and there will be an electrical jolt overhead and a major thriving voice will say, "Paula, this is how you were intended to manage your life". As helpful as that would be for consolation reasons, sadly, it doesn't occur that way. It's significantly more unobtrusive and along these lines, exceptionally not entirely obvious. As a matter of fact, for the majority of us, our motivation and enthusiasm will be looking straight at us but since they don't have fancy odds and ends on them, we might not have taken note!

I'm certain that you have sooner or later thought, " Why am I here? What is my motivation throughout everyday life? What is my obsession? What would be an ideal next step?" These are the absolute most normal inquiries that individuals pose and the most well-known questions that individuals battle with. So we should investigate them a touch more.

How to find purpose -passion in life

What is the purpose?

We spend such a long time looking for it, yet do we try and understand what it implies? I think most of us make reasons to be excessively weighty, excessively strange, and excessively intense! Seeing reason from that perspective can go about as a barricade, as a hindrance.

As I would like to think and from the examination that I've done throughout the course of recent years, I've come to accept that the best and most remarkable definition of design is: Authenticity.
My conviction is that design is tied in with seeing your true self and setting the aim to live such that praises anything it is you find. What's the significance here for you?
Enthusiasm is one more word I believe is in many cases misconstrued with regards to profession and life reasons. Frequently when I work with clients to assist them with finding their interests, they are anticipating that it should be something that they will be fixated on, something that would give them container heaps of energy and make them leap up at 6 am in the first part of the day chomping at the bit to get everything rolling! What I've found for myself actually and for different clients who have found their interests is that energy is a lot milder, it's calmer, you embrace it, you do it for quite a long

time without acknowledging it, there's no show, no ringers, no whistles - just you accomplishing something you love. The most effective way I have found to portray energy is that when you're energetic about something, it seems like a yes.

I accept that every one of us has a reason and a legitimate approach to being and living. Distinguishing, recognizing, and regarding this is maybe the absolute most significant move that blissful individuals make. They carve out opportunities to comprehend what they're here to do and afterward they seek after that with energy and excitement. Or then again, all in all, they find an opportunity to grasp themselves, to interface with their true self, incline toward what feels like a 'yes' (regardless of whether it's frightening) and they set the expectation to live such that they respect themselves.

Without a reason (without being your legitimate self), it's not difficult to get derailed as you carry on with life. It's not difficult to meander and float, achieving pretty much nothing. Be that as it may, with a reason, all that in life appears to get sorted out. To be 'deliberately' signifies you are acting naturally, making every moment count to do, doing what you're great at, and achieving what means a lot to you. It's utilizing your assets of time, energy, and cash on things that you truly care about.

So the fundamental inquiry here I assume is, how would you associate with your real self? How do you have any idea about when you're deliberate? Over the past number of years, I have run over numerous lessons, books, and articles which discuss us having different 'selves'. The idea that reverberated most with me and with most other twenty and thirty-something ladies is the possibility of the 'legitimate self' and 'the social self. To genuinely find your motivation and your interests, you want to get to know your two selves. Allow me to present to you:

The social self is that piece of you that has been impacted by your way of life, your current circumstance, your companions, your family, and society as you have grown up and all through your life. It has trained you to esteem something similar or comparable things to most others in your circle, for example, steady work, being monetarily secure, claiming your own home, meeting an accomplice, having a family, having benefits, caring for your folks - being a 'decent young lady' will we say!

The real self is the piece of you that knows your inclinations for everything; it understands what you appreciate, what you're energetic about, what gives you pleasure, and what you love to do. The valid self realizes that you need to arrange dessert in the café while the social self will tell you not to be a piggy as no other person is having anything! The genuine self is that piece of you that is unconstrained, inquisitive, captivated with the world, and fun-loving.

Having an advanced social self can be an extraordinary resource, notwithstanding, when it is excessively predominant, it can remove us from our genuine self who has all the data that we want to find our actual reason and our actual longings. The allegory I use for this is that the social self is the vehicle yet the bona fide self is the objective. The vehicle could work impeccably yet if we don't have a clue about the objective, it implies we're burning through a ton of time cruising all over around and around.

A great deal of us seldom talk with our internal identities and more often than not we steer our lives in light of the directions of others (who truly do frequently have our wellbeing on a fundamental level) yet who truly have no clue about what we're energetic about and consequently they have no clue about how to assist us with tracking down our motivation. Accordingly, normally, we wind up driving off course.

How can you say whether you're heading on some unacceptable path?

Assuming you feel disengaged with your life/vocation, restless, disappointed, furious, or exhausted then I would risk a reasonable deduction that your two selves aren't functioning admirably together!

Expression of Warning: My recommendation to every individual who is in a task that they are troubled about is to remain where you are until you figure out how to reconnect with your credible self. The justification for this is because the odds are extremely high that you will escape into another work that you could do without and your social self will take the rules much more and advise you to hold your head down, your mouth shut because work should be hard and hopeless.

I'm interested, are your motivation and your interests looking straight at you? Get some margin to incline toward what feels like a 'yes' and you'll begin to realize what your actual cravings are. For the present. This is a central issue so listen cautiously. The vast majority oppose their interests and what they trust their motivation to be because they don't have the assurance that this is what they maintain that they should do for eternity. They don't have a gem ball and they can't take a look at it's the ideal decision. Does this sound natural?

The Impermanence of Purpose

Quite possibly the main thing that I have found out about design is that it changes, similarly to our real self changes. What our identity is changing. At various places in our lives, there will be various things that mean a lot to us. We change, develop and foster in light of our encounters throughout everyday life and our vocations. We're continuously changing and learning new things, shaping novel thoughts regarding what's conceivable. For instance, when I was mulling over my motivation to work with ladies in their 20s and 30s, it was looking straight at me;

however I didn't know whether it was the best decision. I wavered, I re-thought myself and I questioned because consistently I thought, I will not have the option to in any case work with that bunch when I'm more seasoned. I thought, "When I'm advanced in like in my fifties, nobody in their 20s will need to work with me. That can't be correct." However, at that point, I discovered that my motivation could change. However long I had the option to associate with my valid self and understand what 'yes' felt like, I'd continuously have the option to track down my new reason if I grew out of the former one.

CHAPTER TWO

PILLARS OF HEALTH

Consistently new investigations about diet, way of life, and wellbeing spring up. Staying aware of the furthest down-the-line discoveries can be overpowering, particularly when new examinations go against the old. Is espresso positive or negative for you? Will a glass of red wine around evening time safeguard your heart, or increment your gamble of cancer? Exercise is perfect for you — yet how much do you truly need?

Has your primary care physician at any point recommended you figure out more, eat better, cut down on pressure, or hit the hay before? You're in good company. Specialists broadly consider workout, great nourishment, unwinding, and rest urgently to solid living. Furthermore, your Medicare plan might have the option to assist you with consolidating these alleged "four points of support" of good well-being into your day-to-day everyday practice.

As a general rule, accomplishing great well-being works best on the off chance that you improve on your methodology and disregard all the commotion. What I've realized, both in medication and throughout everyday life, is that well-being isn't muddled. That zeroing in on four essential primary parts of wellbeing dependably makes prosperity, expanded energy, and euphoria. My four mainstays of well-being are a legitimate eating regimen, a sound dynamic way of life, quality rest, and association with others. These four points of support are the establishment for becoming as sound, lively, and vivacious as you can be.

Every pillar is similarly significant. You can't practice a terrible eating routine or interface happily with others when you're depleted and restless. I can vouch for the strength of these five pillars since I'm in better shape and more joyful in my fifties than I was in my twenties or thirties. In any case, we as a whole are human. Zeroing in similarly on every one of the four of the mainstays of wellbeing all the time isn't practical for a great many people.

Fortunately, it doesn't make any difference which support point you start with. Research shows that individuals who make solid propensities in a single part of their life wind up making sound propensities in different regions, as well. Individuals make some simpler memories adhering to their objectives when they have prepared, so plan. Start with the support point that persuades you the most, make substantial objectives, and reliably make a move.

CHAPTER THREE

Pillar One: Healthy Food

I can't imagine a solitary ongoing sickness that isn't effectively impacted by diet. Now and again, dietary systems can switch illnesses. The food varieties you eat are the premise of long haul wellbeing. What's more, the method for eating smart for life is to underline plants and solid proteins. That incorporates entire grains, natural products, vegetables, vegetables (like beans), nuts, and sound oils like additional virgin olive oil or avocado oil.

Two renowned eating regimens that observe these rules incorporate the Mediterranean eating routine and the DASH diet. The two eating regimens are plentiful in fiber, nutrients, and minerals that assist with keeping up with sound pulse and lipids, bring down the gamble of diabetes and coronary illness and keep up with solid weight and energy. Besides, these sorts of plant-based counts calories underscore foods grown from the ground and are stacked with wellbeing-advancing flavonoids, cell reinforcements, and polyphenols that significantly affect wellbeing. For example, one survey of 16 unique examinations that incorporated north of 460,000 grown-ups found that flavonoid consumption altogether safeguarded against cardiovascular infection and mortality.

Sound fats are a vital piece of such eating regimens and incorporate Omega-3 unsaturated fats from fish tight as can be and salmon, from nuts like pecans and almonds, and oils like extra-virgin olive oil and avocado oil,and others.

The uplifting news about plant-driven consume fewer calories is that they will more often than not be antacid. A soluble eating routine stresses vegetables, organic products, and drinking bunches of water while decreasing refined carbs, liquor, meat, and exceptionally handled food. They are known to work on general wellbeing, assist with lessening weight, and further develop life span.

A solid and even eating regimen not just assists your body with performing better, but it likewise advances sound cerebrum capability. At the point when you eat steadily, your body performs better as well as by and large you feel significantly improved. At the point when you feel better, it can enormously emphatically influence your psychological state. You are bound to deal with possibly unpleasant circumstances better when you are feeling better and your psyche is free as a bird. On the contrary side of that, eating awful food varieties can prompt you not to feel too which can antagonistically affect your general emotional wellness and prosperity.

Thus, what precisely is it that plays the biggest element with regards to eating fewer carbs and generally speaking emotional well-being? All things considered, research says everything comes down to destroying wellbeing. Eating quality food varieties advance great stomach microbes which assist with general stomach wellbeing. Unfortunate stomach well-being has been displayed to have an immediate connection with despondency and uneasiness. Consolidating food sources that are high in collagen, fiber, and omega-3 unsaturated fats can assist with further developing your stomach microscopic organisms as well as your general state of mind too.

CHAPTER FOUR

Pillar Two: Movement

Our bodies were destined to move. Notably, an inactive way of life is a gamble factor for a large number of ongoing infirmities, including coronary illness, diabetes, hypertension, corpulence, gloom, osteoporosis, and osteoarthritis. Truth be told, expanded degrees of actual work and wellness are related to a lower hazard of mortality for any reason.

In any case, don't think you need to be a Type An overachiever to receive all the well-being rewards. Moderate activity likewise makes a difference. Assuming you are respectably genuinely dynamic somewhere around three hours out of every week, you can bring down your gamble of passing on by

27%. The latest rules, distributed by the US Department of Health and Human Services (HHS) in 2018 state that the ideal measure of action is 150 to 300 minutes of moderate-force vigorous activity each week. This action can be persistent or in short, explodes. Ten minutes several times each day or 30 minutes five days seven days will get you to that 150 minutes out of every week limit.

Moderate movement implies you're practicing sufficiently hard to raise your pulse and start to perspire. Models incorporate lively strolling, bicycling, cultivating, moving, water high impact exercise, kayaking, or even golf for however long you're doing them enthusiastically enough. You can likewise wear a pedometer, to stroll 10,000 stages every day. Moderate force on a pedometer is 3,900 stages in 30 minutes or less.

Practice influences your different support points. For example, active work assists you with resting better and works on your mindset. Furthermore, just to provide you with a thought of how strong actual work is, a recent report in the lofty diary The Lancet, found that not moving enough can be as risky to wellbeing as smoking. Physical latency prompts 5.3 million passings a year all over the planet, and smoking causes around 5 million passings.

What's more, assuming you favor strolling, concentrates on the show that all you want are 7000-7500 stages each day to diminish the gamble of passing on by 50-70%.

CHAPTER FIVE

Pillar Three: Sleep

We as a whole realize that rest is fundamental for endurance and that rest is the point at which the body and mind fix. During rest, your mind sends waste and poisons out of the phones and acquires supplements, which then, at that point, recharge the phones. While resting your cerebrum scrubs itself up to multiple times quicker than when conscious. Unfortunate rest expands your gamble of stroke, coronary failure, an overabundance of weight, and powerless bones. Unfortunate rest likewise is related to a lower cortisol arousing reaction (CAR), which leads you to be too tired and can increase irritation. That is the spike in the emission of cortisol, a significant chemical that readies your body for the requests of the day.Quality rest is on the downfall, in any case. We rested 25%, not as much as people did quite a while back. One out of five grown-ups rests under 6.5 hours an evening. The ideal measure of rest for a great many people is around 8 hours per night. The people who consistently rest under 6 hours or more than9 hours are not as solid.

To rest soundly, attempt to switch off the 'radiant blue' screens two hours before sleep time. They can upset melatonin cycles. Try not to nibble late around evening time. Attempt a quiet contemplation application or music. Scrub down. Indeed, even weighted covers have been displayed to further develop rest.

An ordinary and sound rest plan is a vital part of both mental and actual well-being. A decent night's rest can go far with regards to feeling quite a bit better and having a useful day. Being very much rested can likewise assist you with being stronger while managing pressure or tension that could spring up during a given day.

CHAPTER SIX

Pillar four: Connection

To wrap things up, remain associated with others, from partners to companions to family. We are social animal groups, and association sustains our brains and spirits. Association assists us with moving into a parasympathetic "quiet and interface" mode, a mode where we likewise rest, fix, and summary.

What's more, make a point to interface with yourself. That can mean requiring some investment for things you love. Reflecting. Taking care of yourself is like getting yourself finished with your hands and feet. Furthermore, since such a large number of individuals battle with keeping up with solid limits and endure the side effects, ensuring you're not overcommitted is essential. Since when you're fatigued by being pulled in an excessive number of headings, you can't deal with yourself. You wind up feeling overstretched, overpowered, and angry.

If you're uncertain about whether or not you have sound limits, pose yourself this inquiry. Do you feel sucked dry by the entirety of your responsibilities? Then you're experiencing what I call "Yes disorder" and now is the right time to roll out certain improvements.

Indeed Syndrome is the tendency to say OK again and again and to an excessive number of things. Indeed Syndrome is much of the time the consequence of needing to be an accommodating person. Of feeling that others' requirements are a higher priority than your own. Indeed Syndrome is a certain method for encountering burnout.

Be that as it may, don't worry because the fix to Yes Syndrome is basic. Say No. Express No to those things that don't serve you. Say No when you hear your inward voice say, "I ought to say OK, however, I truly don't have any desire to."

What I've found in my work with a large number of individuals is that time and again individuals are enduring Yes Syndrome since they don't accept they truly deserve getting what they need. They're not deserving of something else. That they don't merit more. However, you in all actuality do merit more.

And on second thought, associate with others in sound ways. This can incorporate rolling out sound improvements fun by doing it with a companion or chipping in locally.

CHAPTER SEVEN

Pillar Five: Exercise

While we as a whole need that languid day where we don't get off the lounge chair occasionally, doing it a lot can be destructive to both our physical and emotional well-being. Moving our bodies and getting activity can work on your general state of mind, however, it likewise delivers endorphins and enkephalins, the body's regular lighthearted chemicals. Standard activity can increment explicit volumes of cerebrum areas. This can further develop oxygen and supplement conveyance that eventually support cerebrum development. Normal activity has been displayed to battle wretchedness and nervousness.

Day-to-day actual work is urgent; whether it's a proper activity class, yoga or pilates meeting or just strolling or cycling, or even housework. These exercises should turn into a set piece of your everyday daily schedule. While holding back nothing can maybe be a test on the off chance that you are not used to being dynamic every day, you will before long end up stimulated and strengthened which will motivate you to proceed with a customary workout daily practice.

Exercises, for example, yoga shift in style and are intended to concentrate and work on the nature of your breathing to further develop endurance and energy levels, while the delicate musical breathing procedures center more around lessening pressure,to assist with actuating sound rest.

CONCLUSION

The key is to give equivalent consideration to every pillar of health, as disregarding one could affect your capacity to support others. The more we balance the four support points inside our lives, the better our possibilities of feeling better over the long haul and difficult to kill.

www.ingramcontent.com/pod-product-compliance
Lightning Source LLC
LaVergne TN
LVHW052107160826
845678LV00015B/3418

* 9 7 9 8 8 4 7 0 6 4 0 0 2 *